TREASURE

OF

HEALTHY LIFE

Eat Right, Be Bright, Road to Healthy Life

by

JASVIR KAUR

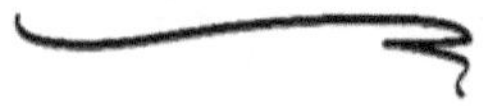

WHY IS THIS BOOK FOR YOU?

We always hear this thought from our elders: Prevention is better than cure, and good health is preferable to a good cure. Everything is changeable in our lives, but the principles of the human body never change. This book helps you adopt these habits in your life so you can stay happy forever. By the way, these habits are required in every man and woman's life, but my book is necessary for those who will be faced with illness. We can break our habits, but we forget it. Once you get the good habit, your brain will force you to do that work. As in the morning, your feet move on to the bathroom for the action of motion. Your mother has instilled this habit from childhood because success comes with health, so it is necessary to know about your health. If you know deeply your health, then you feel how easy life is to survive and achieve success. By reading this book, you can enjoy your life. Study your health with depth. When the sickness of Corona came, people began to have their food habits and health knowledge. Now people have a health interest. There was more health extent in the people before corona. This disease ended a lot of families.

When we look around our surroundings, good health is the greatest gift for those who are sick. The people have no less mental sense, but they are also excuses' if you are ill, then you never become a creator and do not do any work for your community and family. This book tells us how we became fit and healthy to avoid small things in our busy lives and why we are mostly film heroes and heroines because they look very beautiful and smart in their bodies. If you also make your body like that, then the move turns to you. It is not a big question about fitness. It is only to change your small habits.

The future of any human being depends on his health. The future of people's health depends on what can be done to handle health. Health is the fundamental authority of the person, and it should also focus on it to handle it. A good citizen must be in a good society to achieve success in life. In the same way, national prosperity can only come if the people of the country are healthy. Then, the same question in everyone's mind is what health is. Health is the most important subject. In this book, you will read everything about health. Health is a relationship not only with diseases but also with oneself, which is a big subject. If it is called the greatest wealth of human beings, it will not be united.

I know thousands of people who want to know about health but do nothing for health. If someone is aware of this book, I will have fortunately. As a tree looks at so many fruits, some of them are eaten, and some are able to become plants again. And mostly falling and burning. There is also a similar attitude to human health. Those who understand are the best of their lives. Those who do not understand are the victims of the disease. The human mind is the only mind that can show him hell and heaven on earth. It is your mind that can make you rich, healthy, and wealthy. This book will help you with health and fitness information.

Relaxing, resting, and recreation are the most important for a person. The rest of the muscles is a normal way in which organ systems, organs, tissues, cells, and work together to accomplish the complex goal of sustaining life. It is the state of being free from tension and stress. It involves calming the body and can be achieved through various techniques such as deep breathing, meditation, yoga, or simply taking time to rest and unwind. Relaxation is very important for all overall well-being and can help reduce anxiety, improve sleep, and promote a sense of peace and balance. It is essential to incorporate regular relaxation practice into our daily lives to maintain a healthy and balanced.

PREFACE

I start this book with my real small story. I go to my fields once a month to see the crop. On my farm, there is a small pond. There are many small and large birds in the pond. One day, I went into the farms to see how much harm the crop had done after heavy rain. I noticed that the water of the pond was full of fields, and the whole crop had sunk. My mind was very upset to see the submerged crop. I thought that there needed to be a solution to this problem. Then, the Idea came into my brain. Why not put plants around this pond to save from the damage to the farms? Then I thought about planting around the ponds of Safeda and bamboo trees. It was a good jewel. It did not even damage the fields, and the birds also became the residents. But when I went to the field after a month, I noticed that the trees were increasing, but the bamboo plants had stayed the same. Five years later, the white trees fell in the field due to the wind. But bamboo trees, also 15-16 feet high, were standing as they were. They had been fifteen to sixteen feet high in two months. The white trees fell as soon as possible due to the roots on the earth, and the bamboo tree's roots were inside the earth. Even though bamboo trees grow slowly, they are neither broken nor fought. Now, many birds have made the nest on bamboo trees.

Some of our good habits are even bamboo trees, which take time to build but give plenty of pleasure. All of these are good habits in being careful about your health. If this habit is made to be strengthened, we avoid diseases in old age. Our diagnosis increases. Many people in the world are victims of obesity and diseases. Every family seems to have at least one member who tends to be irritable and easily upset. GOD gives us this body as a Gift. We must keep our bodies good and healthy. We go through this book on how we can keep our bodies healthy.

When you are 18 to 20, then you freeze your body for your whole life. Mostly, when we are at this age, we are not aware of our health. So, first of all, we know what health is.

TABLE OF CONTENTS

PART 1: HEALTH...11

    WHAT IS HEALTH 13

    LIVE WITH YOURSELF 17

    HOW TO HELP NERVE ORGAN 21

    BOOST YOUR DEFENCE SYSTEM 23

    OUR IMMUNITY 25

PART 2: HABITS THAT CAN BREAK DOWN YOUR HEALTH 33

    AVOID CLINOPHILIA HABIT 35

    BE AWARE OF ANY TYPES OF DRUGS. 38

    DO EXERCISE EVERY DAY FOR GOOD HEALTH. 45

    HOW MEDITATION AND YOGA KEEP YOU COOL. 49

PART3: NUTRITION 55

    WHAT IS BALANCE DIET. 57

    MINERALS AND VITAMINS 59

    PROTEIN IN DIET. 61

    WATER INTAKE OR DRINKING WATER. 66

PART 4: WORKING HABITS 73

    WHY WORKING HABITS? 75

    GARDENING 77

    READ GOOD BOOKS. 78

    CONTROL YOUR WEIGHT. 80

    REDUCE STRESS 81

DISCLAIMER 85

MAY I ASK YOU A FAVOR? 87

PART 1: HEALTH

Along Life's Pathway

WHAT IS HEALTH

Health is that treasure, the key to guarding to has given us himself. It is expected that those who have good health will take full care of it. So that this treasure will not go away from his hands, he should be fully informed of the fulfillment of this Order; fitness makes you feel a positive attitude to work. Remaining the main sign of health without being stopped and without tiredness, keep working. Health is not limited to only disease-free but instead to living-awake health.

It is a life check-in itself. The world will rise to many diseases in the days to come. There is also a big contribution to environmental changes in our health. But we are all responsible for these environmental changes. Now, health experts think that your health is your responsibility. Safety of the environment and understanding others are our responsibility.

Where we live, what is our occupation, what do we eat, which water do we drink, and what are our thoughts? All these aspects are responsible for our health. The person's body is weak; he can never take determination. Health is the name of physical, mental, emotional, and social strength. Good health helps people to build strength. Health means people are filled with enthusiasm. An enthusiastic man is different from a crowd of people. Actually, health is also the key to success, education, citizenship, and happy life.

Dimensions of Health

There are three Dimensions of health-1-Physically, 2-mentally, 3-socially.

But it is also felt that some other dimensions are related to health, like emotional, spiritual, nutritional, environmental, and educational.

Curative and Preventive

Education

Nutritional

Emotional

Physical

Mental

Social

Environmental

Vocational

Spiritual

Physical Dimensions- Physical Dimension means the whole physically and mentally; all parts of the body are included in it. External means height, weight, color, form, Nayan mint, strong physical organs, beautiful physical structure, and efficiency of work. The inside means all internal systems like the Digestive system, blood circulation system, respiratory system, and sticky cell system. Working with all physical systems.

Mental Dimensions: Mental health is related to everyone's emotional relations. Because of this relationship, a human being behaves in love with others. Sertorius has affected the mental nature that the balance around him is dependent. It is affected by internal and external. Our brain has three types of glands that release four types of hormones. The names of those hormones are Dopamine, serotonin, oxytocin, and endorphin. Most people do not know about these Harmon, but some people know about them and underestimate the pows. Hormones play a huge role in everyone's life, and all of us, in our daily routine and food habits, make some small and simple changes. Balancing these happy hormones can increase your peace and happiness level manifold. This increases your creativity, productivity, and energy level, and you can make a big positive change in your relationship in a very short time. And by staying motivated every moment, you can fill life with happiness. And what are things that you can keep in mind? The brain communicates with every part of the body at every moment. At the same time, he keeps on releasing such special hormones, which is a special remote system for the body of the brain. It is also called a hormone or chemical of reward, which is actually a neurotransmitter. Actually, whenever you complete a task or achieve a goal, the brain releases dopamine as a reward that makes you feel happy. That is, you get pleasure from dopamine released by the brain. So that you are motivated to do work again and again.

Social Dimensions- The social dimension of health refers to our ability to make and maintain meaningful relationships with others. Good social health includes not only having relationships but behaving appropriately within them and maintaining socially acceptable standards. The basic social unit of relationships is the family, and these relationships impact a person's life the most. Other key relationships are close friends, social networks, teachers, and youth leaders. Sometimes, we think that we have knowledge of everything, and others are foolish and do not help others. But when we are alone, then we really, what is socialism.

I met an army man's family. The whole family was very intelligent, but they did not have any friends in their street. There are six members in the family. Only two people knew about car driving. One day, one of them fell sick, and they both were drivers going out of their homes, and no one came to them for their help. My home was near them. I reached out to them for their help as humanity. I lifted them and was admitted to the hospital. A few days later, when they were fine, they came to my home to thank me for this help. I told them that there was no need for thanks. It's my duty as humanity. They feel shy because they never have someone's help. But they said to me, if any social help is needed, tell us it is necessary. Thus, they found out that living in society is very important to socialize.

Environmental Dimension: A person's internal environment and surroundings represent his health level. Environment is an important part of health. How high is the level of life? This is known only for the cleaning of the house and street. The surrounding cleansing shows a beautiful and healthy style of life. If a person has a mental illness, then first, he put the dirtiness around him. He will spare things in his house. Will also spare his hair. You have to see that the mad people have their hair separated. Their clothes were filled with dirt.

LIVE WITH YOURSELF

Everyone in this world needs the help of others. Become a good supporter of your family, friends, and others who need your help. Nerve problems are so common in humans. Every normal person is affected by nervous problems, even those who always look calm and relaxed. After the age of +45, every person who never cares for themself is badly ill.

Every family has one member who has a nerve problem and is upset with himself. Some of them are never able to come and go anywhere. Their moods often change very suddenly. Everyone can always be sour about how they will react and how you can help those people. If you ignore them, then it is your big mistake. Mostly, their problem arises from hidden fears, while he knows that he cannot do anything about them.

My mother is also about to get this problem too late. When she began bowing and walking, I asked my mother about this problem, and she started weeping and telling me. I took him to the doctor and gave her treatment. Similarly, many other people are suffering from nervous problems.

How it would be wonderful if we had some magic formula, perhaps eating some drugs and putting an injection, that would solve the problem. Only by learning and understanding ourselves.

Most people come to the doctor when this problem calculates other complaints together.

Some suffer in silence because no one can understand them, not even their family.

Understand your near and dear

Understand your family members, friends, and others around you because it is so easy to criticize and misunderstand others. Sometimes, you also take the probe but still keep talking to be afraid. In this case, we should talk to him closely. And he should get treatment if we can understand others so that God is blessed upon us. Because the nerve problem can convert to cancer at any time, it must be treated as soon as possible.

This is not affected by this problem; sometimes they take a serious sickness and some tragedy to make them merciful towards others who are in trouble, socially their relatives and dear friends. In the world, many people who are the most famous are nervous.

When things are not working according to them, they have serious nerve stress. Some of them suffer from Frome headaches. They are a good service provider for society. They are those people who work for others. And we must cheer them up. If you are these types, then you are in good company. If you have these qualities and you put them to work, then you do something special to change in life. If

you can solve your emotional problem by understanding something about yourself, then you are in a good direction. Life is very short; do not disappoint anyone who is doing good. If you do not do good for others, then don't disturb those who are doing well for others. Those who are suffering from mental breakdowns actually don't know about the real joy of living. Be thankful to God; you are not in them.

Some other points to understand others

1- Listen actively; Pay attention to what others are saying and give them your full focus without interrupting or thinking about your response.

2- Show empathy; -Try to understand and share the feelings of others and acknowledge their emotions without any judgment.

3- Ask questions; -Show genuine interest in others by asking open-ended questions to learn more about their experiences.

4- Be patient -Be patient and give others the time and space to express themselves without any fear.

5- Be minded; -talk to them and be willing to consider different viewpoints and their opinions.

6- Respect boundaries; Respect the personal space and boundaries of others during conversations.

7- Pay attention to nonverbal cues; observe body language, facial expressions, and tone of voice to understand the emotions of others better.

8- Seek common ground: Look for shared interests or experiences that can help you connect with others on a deeper level.

9- Offer support -Be there for others in times of need and offer your support and encouragement when they are facing troubles.

10- Practice active communication; -Clearly express your thoughts and feelings while also being receptive to the thoughts and feelings of others in order to foster mutual understanding.

In view of the above, we can reach out to close others.

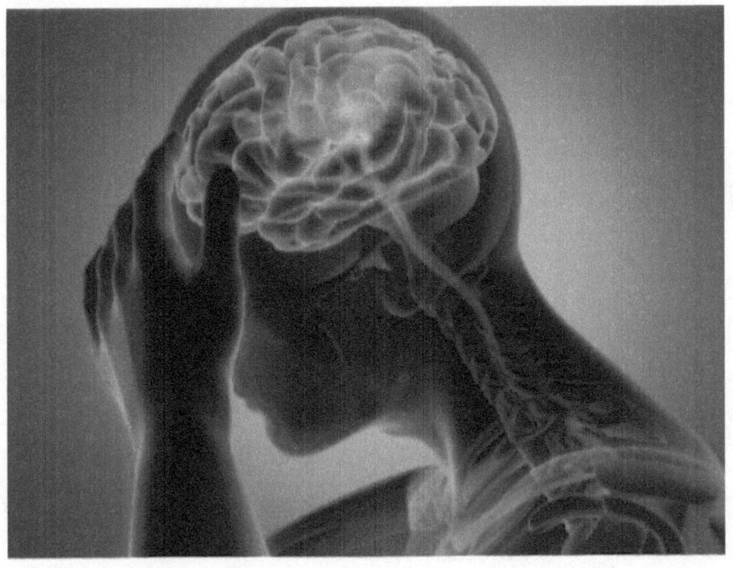

HOW TO HELP NERVE ORGAN

The nervous system is the organ system responsible for sending and receiving signals throughout the body. It includes the brain, spinal cord, and a network of nerves that transmit electrical impulses to and from different parts of the body. The nervous system controls everything, From basic body functions like breathing and heart rate to more complex processes like thinking, feeling, and moving.

Nerves to be cause all body trouble. They are the most remarkable organs in our body. When babies are born, they have millions of nerves carried with them. The baby could not digest his food without nerves. Every movement of the newborn baby, cry, breathe depends on the nervous system. Our growth and development totally depend on our nerves.

As a human being, we can make our decisions. Health is often the result of a nervous system that is pushed beyond its normal limits of endurance. How to go away without any difficulty depends on our family background.

Some things happen in our childhood that we are suffering from, and that was not in our control, but some people keep on feeling sick forever.

This is mostly due to their bad habits. Also known as everything, everything becomes unknown. We should not have any excuse to understand our nervous system.

Some nervous people enjoy being sick. It is known to see them that they have dramatic symptoms. These only draw special attention to themselves. But this enjoyment pays a heavy price. Most nervous people want to get well soon. They want good health to enjoy.

This book has all the rules that are required for good health. Remember that the excuses will only allow you to succeed if you make money and sustain health.

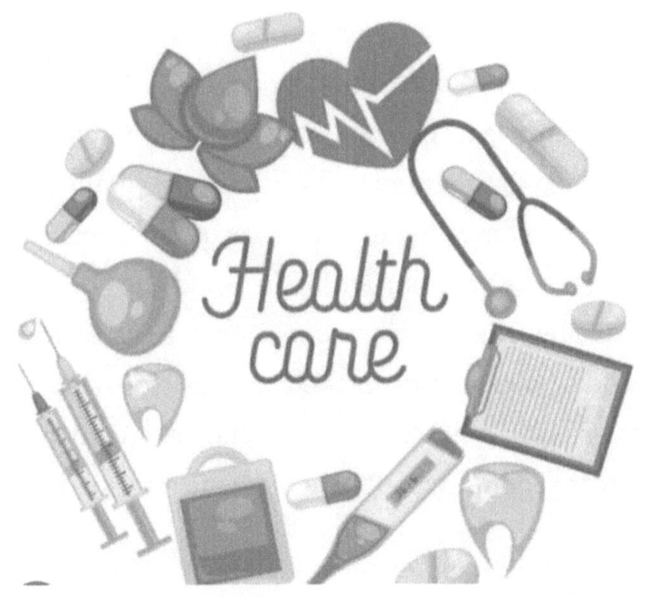

BOOST YOUR DEFENCE SYSTEM

The body defense System works exactly as the army works on the borders to save the country. If we want our bodies to look different from other people, then we have to do a different task than others. It will be exactly as the enemy attaches out of the outside, and we respond hardly. Germs are everywhere present in our environment. These are not made of any hard things like iron and plastic. It entered our bodies anywhere. If our internal defense system is strong, it means when your body's army is strong, then any outsider enemies cannot disturb your internal properties. Germs are our enemies; we will have to take our health to protect them.

In this protection system, the main defense is our skin. Our skin can resist the penetration of germs into the underlying tissues. Secondly, our white blood cells, which are called leukocytes, move from place to place in our body and have the capacity to kill germs and viruses and even totally clean them. When we don't care to build a strong army, it means defense; many germs destroy our antibodies, and they do not destroy the germs but can identify them as open to diversion. When a new kind of germ enters the body and causes sickness like the coronavirus or chicken pox, antibodies are made in such quantity that some are left over after the attacker is uprooted.

Whenever the skin is a very strong barrier against the raid of germs into the internal tissues, but once it is broken, germs attack the naked tissues, damage parts of the skin, and become infected. When germs close the eyes, then you cannot stop infection because the membranes of the eyes are the common entry points of germs and are constantly exposed to the environment. Bacteria, viruses, and pathogens can come easily into contact with the eyes, leading to infections such as pink eyes or other eye infections. It is important to practice good hygiene. Avoid touching the eyes with dirty hands and seek medical attention if you suspect an eye infection to prevent the spread of the infection and protect your overall health.

After skin and eyes, the next most important organ of our body is NOSE. It filters the air; a person breathes as it enters the body. It has an army team as a hair, which is located at the entrance to the nostrils. The large dust particulars cannot land in it with germs. When coronaviruses spread all over the world, the Nose is the only organ that every person in the world covers because the membranes that line the nose and other air passengers are constantly covered with mucus; it controls the air that moves toward the lungs.

The next organ is our mouth, which is the cause of infection; if we do not care about our food and personal sagenite food, which enters the mouth, we may be infected with germs, but we have stopped its supply. Other facilities for destroying the germs as they entered with the food depended upon the disastrous action of the baby's gastric juice. This badly affects the stomach. If you know about your body's protective system, then you are able to protect your body from diseases

OUR IMMUNITY

Our immunity refers to the body's ability to resist and fight infections and diseases. It is a complex system that involves cells, proteins, and organs working together to defend the body against harmful bacteria, viruses, and other harmful parasites, which are bad for our body. The immune system recognizes and responds to unknown possibilities, making an immune response to eliminate them from the body. This can include the production of antibodies, the activation of immune cells, and the development of immunological memory to provide long-term protection against specific pathogens. A strong immune system is essential for maintaining overall health and preventing illness.

Artificial Immunization

Vaccination, also known as artificial immunization, works by introducing a weakened or inactive form of a pathogen [such as a virus or bacteria] into the body. This stimulates the immune system to produce antibodies and activate immune cells without causing the actual disease.

Once the immune system has been exposed to the weakened or inactive pathogen, it develops immunological memory, which allows it to recognize and respond more effectively if the body is later exposed to the actual, harmful form of the bacteria. This provides long-term protection against the disease.

Vaccines are designed to mimic natural infections and help the body develop immunity without causing illness. They have been instrumental in controlling and eradicating many infectious diseases and have significantly reduced the incidence of serious illnesses and deaths worldwide.

We can be very thankful for the body to have several mechanisms by which our resistance to disease is maintained, as our protective provisions are marvelous. Their degree of efficiency depends upon one's state of health. Each person must make sure that they follow a way of life that promotes physical fitness and makes their body's defenses most effective.

Sometimes accidents occur in life, which are difficult to get out of. Every part of the world continues to happen. It is warming in many countries, and diuretics and earthquakes. How much innocence and financial loss of every day in these events. In it, many people are victims of mental suffering. Rest and recreation can only expel one from this situation.

Nothing in the world is bigger than human confidence. If you think deeply, the biggest trouble begins to small with your confidence. When you think that you are alone, then do some day rest and relax your muscles, take a deep breath, and think that nothing lives forever in the world. If no one has been in the world, if you have been, then anything of nature, such as the birds, animals, or land, can be made up for your own. It can be best fun to take care of others. Planting, gardening, dancing, singing, book reading, and many more activities are the most common, which are to give you relief from brain fatigue. Doing those things that you love helps reduce stress, promote relaxation, and make time for activities that bring you joy.

Avoid stressful things

If some things happen that are not in your control, then why do you get any stress, and which is in your control, then why worry? The efficiency of the body is badly affected when you feel unnecessary stress. When you think it is a very difficult task for me, then take others to help those who are experts in those things. Everyone is only an expert in some things. Every time, we need someone, and these needs are making a bond with others.

If you should live a healthy lifestyle, then be simple. Which work should you do? You need to plan for your work with greater efficiency and study better methods of your work.do some work daily to create things like growing some plants around your house. The development of happy hormones depends on proper relaxation. It would be best if you had a proper balance between your body, mind, and soul. It would be best if you also balanced the spiritual, physical, and mental aspects of life.

When we become civilized, we think that our life becomes very easy, but it has many disadvantages. It has upset the balance between our mental, physical, and spiritual life. Because of it, many people had stress, which became the cause of lack of sleep and rest. Modern lifestyle is a very busy lifestyle. No one has time for themselves. So, a hard and fast lifestyle causes a stressful life. The balance of life upset.

Here I tell the story of a man who lives in my village. He has a small piece of land. He gets up early in the morning and does his work in two or three hours; after this, he eats his food and takes a rest. He has four daughters and one son. He has some cows and one buffalo. In the evening, at nearly four o'clock, he and his wife finish their work, and they all eat food collectively, his children and they both, husband and wife. The people of the village think about how he can manage his daughter's marriage and their studies. But he never thinks about it. His thinking is that whoever is born on this earth is bringing his food from God. He said that I would give my child a healthy lifestyle. It will not give them a luxury lifestyle. They will read in government schools. And it will make their life on yourself. Many people tell him that you can make more money, but for what? He answered. He makes his life very easy. He never listens to anyone's suggestions. But most people never like this farmer.

Excessive nervous and muscular stress causes anxiety or pain. Especially for those people who are worried about responsibility, the condition of our nervous system is disturbed, which causes indigestion, acidic stomach, constipation, and nervous failure. Many people don't do any exercise in their tensions. Even if people are civilians, like doctors, teachers, engineers, business people, and politicians, they also do not pay attention to their fitness.

Whether you are civilized or not, your health is the most important part of life. The demand of civilized life is not only to mess with disease but also to cut down recreation. The solution to this problem is that you only have to reduce the reasons that give you tension or stress. This way, you can raise the happiness of your living.

Include Recreation in your life

My friend is in England. She says that husband and wife meet once a week. Working is reduced to dependence on each other. But the conversations with each other have been less. With this situation, the distance increases between us. Now, we meet each other like strangers. The children also remain silent. So, I told them that the solution is also with you. On the holiday, you all get out of the house. Sit together all in a day of the week and eat together. Which activity do you get satisfaction from?

There will be many other families like this who suffer from this situation. We can get out of many situations by adding entertainment to our lives. It can be in many ways.

1- CommunityRrecreation
2- Family Recreation
3- Institutional Recreation
4- Therapeutic Recreation
5- Commercial Recreation

It is not necessary to go to another country or any outside state to entertain. It is done with the people of your village or street, who can be involved in their daily life activities. It is the basic need of humans.

Recreation plays a big role in human happiness. There is a big bond between health and recreation. It takes a human being away from diseases; it also can heal people. This causes a decrease in crimes and is also characterized. Recreation encourages disappointing people.

During the war, a military man lost his leg. He became very frustrated with his life. His wife was a very intelligent woman. She took him to a park by seating him in a wheelchair every day. He was happy to see children play in the park. Some men and women who walked in the park gossiped with him. The doctor told his wife that recovery of his leg would be very soon. And soon we put an artificial leg of it. Now, he could walk like a commoner. All this happened because of the entertainment. So, recreation plays a big role in our lost life.

In the entire creation, the human mind is the most delicate thing., and the most sensitive device. By placing it cool and healthy, it can be taken forward with unbelievable success. But if you don't care if you get losses. Keep your brain fit in every obstacle in life. Always keep encouraging your brain. I will do this work very well. This philosophy works like magic for your mind. When you keep your mind stress-free, then the better way to work in your mind begins to come on.

Always keep away from negative people. They always prevent you from proceeding. Developing your thinking means moving forward to your success. If you want to be an important person, leave your brain open. Whenever you are doing some work, do it from your heart. Make a routine to do everything. It makes your life stress-free.

PART 2: HABITS THAT CAN BREAK DOWN YOUR HEALTH

AVOID CLINOPHILIA HABIT

Laziness is a state of unwillingness to exert effort or energy. It can manifest as a lack of motivation, procrastination, or the action of delaying, or a desire to avoid work and responsibilities. While everyone experiences moments of laziness from time to time, chronic laziness can have negative impacts on a person's personal and professional life.

There are many potential causes of laziness, including psychological factors such as depression or anxiety, physical factors such as fatigue or illness, and environmental factors such as a lack of motivation or moral support. Overcoming laziness often requires self-reflection, goal-setting, and developing healthy habits and routines.

It is important to address laziness in a compassionate and understanding manner, as it may be a symptom of underlying issues that need to be addressed. Seeking support from friends, family, or mental health professionals can be helpful in overcoming chronic laziness and building a more fulfilling and productive.

Avoid Laziness – To see the sunrise is a sign of luck or fortune. In this high-speed life, we sleep late at night and get up in the morning to lie down. You are busy no matter how much you live at work. But it would be best if you went to sleep until 11 o'clock. And should get up early in the morning. The morning time is the most energetic. During this time, you should do work that is related to your body and mind. Like yoga, exercise, and if you are a writer or player, then it is the priciest time for you. But if the modern-time people have left up getting up early in the morning. Students keep studying until night and go to sleep in the morning. But you don't know that a sleeping hormone is most important for your health and brain.

Leave your mobile phone when you go to sleep. Try to avoid using your mobile phone at the dining table or when you are sitting with your family. Sometimes, we sit in the family, still the mobile phone in our hands. In today's times, the mobile has become their own, relations are not important.

One of my friends who has a government job is a very lazy person. When it's time to work, he starts to eat; when the time is for having food, then he starts work. He lay on the bed in the evening and watched reel on Instagram. His family members were very disturbing to him. His body structure becomes like a sumo Palawan, but he never cares about it. His children are very fad up from him. In the morning, he gets up late from bed and starts quarreling with his wife. Where are my clothes? You don't care about me; I will leave you and arrange one servant to care for myself, etc. One day, His wife came to his workplace by heart from him. She asked all his friends to improve his habits. Otherwise, our family will be malicious. But he did not leave his bad habits on the college suggestions. After a few days, the massage came to the office, and he died due to a heart attack in the middle of the night. After his death, the government was given to his wife his job. This story tells us the moral that don't play with your health with your bad habits. There are many more stories in our social curriculum. Born on the earth as a human being, so live like humans, not like animals.

You have to make an effort for him before doing any work. This is the principal law of nature: none of the things themselves are beginning, neither are there any widening devices that deal with your essential work as soon as you make a pinch as you have to hit her lever before you get a car gear. This theory is also about your mind. The first brain will be to be addicted to the right habits. This will work very well for you.

Make your daily routine work which you do, like,

1- Get out of bed early in the morning.

2- Give thanks to God for one new morning.

3- Go out for a morning walk.

4- brush your teeth.

5- Take a bath.

6- Take a cup of coffee or tea.

7- Eat your breakfast.

8- Wear your clothes and get ready.

9- Take your things for your work.

10- Start your work with full energy.

Start with small changes in your behavior, and you find that you have a big change in your habits. If you see that to convince your mind to do small things on a daily basis, you will have great success in changing your bad habits, and you will succeed in your goal in life. You think that if you make your habits good, then you help the people around you because they look to you and try to become like you.

BE AWARE OF ANY TYPES OF DRUGS.

Meaning of drugs- Which thing stimulates a person mentally and physically is called drugs. It is used as a helper to improve work efficiency. This is impressed on the tissues as they enter the person. Usually, it is understood that drugs work miraculously in increasing the efficiency of the person. The internal system of each person is different.

One drug can be poisoned for the other person. Drugs may also be dangerous to improve work efficiency and the advantages of comfort. In the same way, medicine can be miraculous for some and poisonous for others.

Why People Use Drug

1- Unemployment- It is the main reason for unemployment for young and adult people. Low employment for the youth, they feel emptiness around their surroundings. They become disappointed by this and get drugs.

2- Lack of occupational education

3- Unsuccessfulness: a person does not have any success in his aim, then he starts taking drugs.

4- Due to friend effects in school and college, friends compel each other to get drugs.

5- Sails of unfair medicine or drugs- Each place must ban unfair drugs and medicines.

6- Spending more than your income. A person's income is less, and his expenditure is more than his income, and he gets depressed and takes the drug.

7- Minimizing physical labor modernization, most people do not want to do hard work; they think it is not their duty.

8- Development of new drugs: people are attracted to them and want to see their taste by seeing new drugs.

9- Irresponsibility a child is in his childhood; parents do not tell them to do their homework. Children become irresponsible when they become adults, and they can't do any hard work, and the habit of free living makes them lazy. And he takes the drugs.

10- Less education about the work.

11- Drugs for poor people are a source of recreation.

12- Preparation of examination- Students get drugs during the preparation of the exam.

13- Sportspeople take drugs to improve in games and to win the games.

14- To minimize physical fatigue.

15- For pain relief, drugs like ibuprofen, acetaminophen, and aspirin are commonly used to relieve pain and reduce inflammation.

16- Antibiotics- These drugs are used to treat bacterial infections and prevent the spread of harmful bacteria in the body.

17- Blood thinner drugs like warfarin and heparin are used to prevent blood clots and reduce heat stroke and heart attack.

18- Insulin- This hormone is used to treat diabetes by regulating blood sugar levels in the body.

19- Chemotherapy drugs- These medications are used to treat cancer cells.

20- Steroids- These drugs are used to reduce inflammation and suppress the immune system in conditions like asthma and arthritis

Bad Effects of Drugs

1- Addiction-Drugs can cause physical and psychological dependence, leading to addiction and compulsive drug-seeking behavior.

2- Overdose- Taking too much of a drug can lead to overdose, which can be fatal.

3- Liver damage- Some drugs, especially those containing acetaminophen, can cause liver damage with long-term use or in high doses.

4- Kidney damage- Certain drugs can cause kidney damage and impair kidney function.

5- Cardiovascular problems- Some drugs can increase the risk of heart attack, stroke, and other cardiovascular issues.

6- Respiratory problems- Drug abuse can lead to respiratory issues, including difficulty breathing and lung damage.

7- Mental health issues- Drug abuse can exacerbate or cause mental health disorders such as anxiety, depression, and psychosis.

8- Memory loss- long-time drug habit can damage your brain functions and lead to memory loss.

9- Increased risk of infectious diseases- Dengue can increase the risk of contracting infectious diseases such as HIV and hepatitis through needle sharing and risky behaviors.

10- Congenital disabilities- Using the drugs during pregnancy can cause congenital disabilities and development issues in the baby.

11- Relationship problems- Drug abuse can strain relationships with family, friends, and romantic partners.

12- Impaired judgment- Drugs can impair judgment and decision-making, leading to risky behaviors and accidents.

13- Legal issues- Drugs can create legal problems, including arrests and criminal charges.

14- Financial problems- Drug addiction can lead to financial problems due to the cost of obtaining drugs and the inability to hold down a job.

15- Social isolation- Drug abuse can lead to social isolation and withdrawal from friends and family.

16- Physical health problems use can increase health issues, including malnutrition, weight loss, and chronic illnesses.

17- Risky behavior- Drug abuse can cause risky behaviors such as unsafe sex, driving under the influence, and criminal activities.

18- Withdrawal symptoms- Stopping certain drugs can lead to withdrawal symptoms, including nausea, vomiting, tremors, and seizures.

19- Less tolerance power- Higher doses of drugs can cause a decrease in tolerance power.

20- Death- In severe cases, drugs can lead to fatal overdoses or long-term health complications that result in death.

A simple treatment for druggy people

1- Please encourage them to seek professional help from therapists and counselors.

2- Providing them with a supportive and non-judgmental environment.

3- Please help them to join a supportive group.

4- Helping them to develop healthy coping mechanisms and stress management techniques.

5- Encouraging them to engage in physical exercise and physical activity.

6- Assisting them in creating a structured daily routine.

7- Providing them with resources for addiction recovery.

8- Please encourage them to practice mindfulness and meditation.

9- Assisting them in finding their hobbies and activities to keep them occupied and motivated.

10- Encouraging them to build strong support and bonds with family.

11- Please help them to find purpose and meaning in their lives.

12- Please help them with self-care and well-being.

13- Helping them to set realistic and achievable goals for their recovery.

14- Providing education on the effects of drugs and benefits of sobriety.

15- Help them find employment or volunteer opportunities to build structure and routine in their lives.

I know a person whose name is Amrit. He had been addicted to heroin for years, but after hitting rock bottom and losing everything he cared about, He decided to seek help. With the help of his family and a rehabilitation program, He was able to overcome his addiction and start a new life. He now works as a counselor at the same rehabilitation center where he found his path to recovery, helping others who are struggling with addiction.

Here another story of an addicted person names Joban Jit. After spending years in and out of prison due to his drug addiction, Joban Jit finally decided he wanted a different life. He entered a rehabilitation program and dedicated himself to his recovery. With the support of his family and newfound friends, he was able to leave drugs and rebuild his life. He now works as a mentor for others who are struggling with addiction, showing them that there is hope for a better future.

DO EXERCISE EVERY DAY FOR GOOD HEALTH

The way food our life is essential in the same exercise should also be a necessary need of our life. The attractive body seems to be all beautiful, but the question is how to protect it.

According to science, all the organs of our body are renewable, only leaving the Cornea of the eyes. When nature gives us a chance to keep the body fresh, why do you lose it? I know a lot of people who put on drugs prioritize exercise. But they do not know how dangerous these drugs are for them. No matter how busy you are, you should only remove fifteen to twenty minutes for exercise every day.

Meenu is always a busy working mom, juggling her career and taking care of her family. She always needed to make time for exercise. After the age of 42, she was suffering from a heart attack; then, she realized the importance of daily exercise for her overall health. She started regular walks and yoga into her daily routine, and she noticed a significant change in her energy level and overall well-being. Now, she makes exercise a necessary part of her daily schedule because she knows that it is essential for her long-term health.

Get used to playing with your children from childhood. This habit will always connect with sports. This will also save us from unnecessary use of phones and computer addiction. He will never be a victim of depression.

After experiencing chronic stress and suspension from his job, Kadim turned to daily exercise as a way to manage his stress level. He started practicing Yoga and exercising regularly. Exercise become a vital part of his daily routine work. He is happy with his work. He felt that his brain had been working better than before. He starts his new business, earns better than before, and maintains a healthy work-life balance. Kadim does daily exercise as a way to take care of his mental and emotional well-being.

Some people are always eating. They always need to think when and how much to eat. They should pay more attention to their calories. You can get better health by controlling your weight. When you are eighteen, control your weight with exercise and freeze your body at eighteen. When you are overweight, then you have to work hard again to get into that shape.

How to ready for exercise in daily routine

1- Set a specific time for exercise – Choose a time of day that works best for you and stick to it. This will help you establish a routine and make it easier to incorporate exercise into your daily routine.

2- Prepare your workout clothes the night before -Lay out your workout clothes the night before so that you can easily slip into them and get started with the necessary energy. Make sure to stay hydrated by drinking water before, during, and after your workout.

3- Fuel your body with a light snack or meal about 1-2 hours before your workout. It provides your body with the necessary energy.

4- Warm-up: Before starting your exercise routine, spend a few minutes doing some cardio or dynamic stretching to warm your body muscles and prepare your body for the workout ahead.

5- Have a plan – Know what types of exercise you will be doing and have a plan in place. Whether it is a specific workout routine, a fitness class, or a run, having a plan will help you stay focused and motivated.

6- Listen to your body – Pay attention to how your body feels and adjust your workout and type if needed. It's important to listen to your body and not push yourself too hard, especially if you are feeling tired or sore.

7- Cool down and stretch – After the workout, take some time to cool down and stretch your muscles. This will help you prevent injury and improve your flexibility.

8- Rest and recover – Allow your body to rest and recover after your workout by getting enough sleep, eating well, and taking rest days as needed.

By following these steps, you can establish a daily routine that will help you prepare for exercise and make it a regular part of your life.

HOW MEDITATION AND YOGA KEEP YOU COOL

Meditation and Yoga can help keep you cool by promoting your relaxation, reducing stress, and improving emotion regulation. Here's how;

1- Stress reduction -Both Meditation and Yoga are effective in reducing stress levels by activating the body's relaxation response. This helps you lower blood pressure, decrease your heart rate, and reduce muscle tension, which can all contribute to a feeling of coolness.

2- Emotional regulation- Regular practice, meditation, and yoga can help improve emotional regulation by increasing self-awareness and mindfulness. This enables individuals to challenge situations with calmness and clarity.

3- Improved Mental clarity- Meditation and yoga can enhance mental clarity and focus to maintain a sense of composure even in the face of stress.

4- Physical cooling – Certain yoga poses and breathing techniques can help cool the body physically, promoting a sense of calm and relaxation.

Overall, both meditation and yoga have been shown to have a positive impact on mental and emotional well-being, helping you stay cool, calm, and collected in the face of your life's challenges.

What is the Meditation

Meditation is a practice that involves training the mind to achieve a state of mental clarity, emotional calmness, and high awareness. It is often used for relaxation to reduce stress. It can help spiritual growth. Meditation can take many forms, but its common goal is to focus attention and reduce the stream of thoughts that may be crowding the mind.

There are various meditation techniques, including mindfulness meditation, loving-kindness meditation, transcendental meditation, and many others techniques. Some common elements of meditation include finding a quiet and comfortable place to sit or lie down, focusing attention on the breath, a mantra, or an object, and gently redirecting the mind back to the focal point when it wanders.

Practicing meditation regularly has been associated with numerous benefits, such as reduced stress, improved emotional well-being, enhanced self-awareness, better concentration, and even physical health benefits. Many people find that meditation helps them to cultivate a sense of inner peace and balance in their lives.

Benefits of Meditation

Meditation offers a range of potential benefits for both mental and physical well-being. Some of the key benefits of meditation may include-

1- Stress reduction – Meditation can help to lower stress levels by promoting relaxation and reducing the production of stress hormones like cortisol.

2- Improved emotional well-being- Regular meditation practice has been linked to reduced symptoms of anxiety, depression, and mood disorders.

3- Enhanced self-awareness – Meditation encourages self-reflection and introspection, leading to a greater understanding of one's thoughts, emotions, and behaviors.

4- Better concentration and focus- Through training the mind to maintain attention on a specific focal point, meditation can improve cognitive function and concentration.

5- Increased mindfulness – Mindfulness meditation, in particular, helps individuals become more present in the moment and develop a nonjudgmental awareness of their experiences.

6- Emotional resilience – Meditation can build emotional resilience, helping individuals cope with difficult situations and manage their reactions to challenging emotions.

7- Enhanced overall well-being – Many people report an overall improvement in their quality of life, feeling more balanced, calm, and content as a result of regular meditation practice.

8- Physical health benefits – Research suggests that meditation may have positive effects on blood pressure, immune function, pain management, and other aspects of physical health.

It's important to note that individual experiences with meditation can vary, and not everyone may experience all of these benefits. However, many people find that incorporating meditation into their daily routine can have a positive impact on their mental and physical health.

There are many stories about the transformative power of meditation. Here are a few that we all know about but don't care about.

The Buddha's Enlightenment

The Buddha's enlightenment, one of the most well-known stories in the history of meditation, is that of Siddhartha

Gautama, who became the Buddha. After years of seeking enlightenment, Siddhartha sat under a bodhi tree. He entered into deep meditation to attain enlightenment and a deep understanding of the nature of suffering and the path to liberation.

The Power of Meditation

Jon Kabat-Zinn, a renowned meditation teacher, introduced mindfulness meditation to Western medicine in the 1970s. He developed the Mindfulness-Based Stress Reduction [MBSR]program, which has since helped countless individuals cope with chronic pain, stress, and illness. The success of MBSR has led to widespread acceptance of mindfulness as a therapeutic tool in healthcare settings.

The Story of Milarepa

Milarepa was a legendary Tibetan yogi and poet who spent years meditation in remote caves in the Himalayas. Through his intense meditation practice, he achieved profound spiritual realization and became a revered figure in Tibetan Buddhism. His life story is often cited as an example of the transformative power of meditation and the potential for inner awakening.

The Impact of Meditation on Children

In recent years, there have been numerous stories of schools and communities implementing meditation programs for children. These initiatives have shown positive effects on children's behavior, emotional regulation, and academic performance. Many educators and parents have shared inspiring stories of how meditation has helped children become more focused, calm, and empathetic.

These stories illustrate the diverse ways in which meditation has impacted individuals and communities throughout history. They highlight the potential for meditation to bring about profound personal growth, healing, and spiritual awakening.

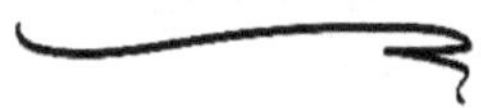

PART3: NUTRITION

WHAT IS BALANCE DIET

Nutrition is the science that makes the knowledge of its uses by food and body. Food provides content that builds and repairs our body tissue, and what we eat affects our health. The right and balanced food prevents the risk of diseases. Balanced food is a way that provides the body with the necessary nutrient elements.

Balanced Diets

Balance diets mean eating the correct type of food and liquid products that provide energy to the body. These can be divided into three types of food.

1-   Growth and Repair food.

2-   Heat and Energy food.

3-   Body Regulators.

1- **Growth and Repair Food** – Foods that are important for growth and repair include those that are rich in protein, healthy fats, vitamins, and minerals. Protein is essential for building and repairing tissues in the body, so foods like lean meats, poultry, fish, eggs, dairy products, legumes, and nuts are important sources of proteins. Healthy fats, such as those found in avocados, nuts, seeds, and olive oil, are also important for growth and repair as they provide energy and help the body absorb essential vitamins.

2- **Heat and Energy food** – The idea of foods that provide the body with a high level of energy or generate heat within the body. This concept is commonly found in traditional or their effects on the body. In many traditional systems of medicine, such as Ayurveda or traditional Chinese medicine, foods are classified based on their energetic properties, which can include their effects on the body temperature and energy levels. In a broader sense, from a nutritional perspective, foods that are often associated with providing '' heat and energy' 'are those that are rich in macronutrients, particularly carbohydrates, which are a primary source of energy for the body, as they are broken down into glucose, which fuels our cells. Foods high in complex carbohydrates, such as whole grains, legumes, and starchy vegetables, are often considered to be good sources of sustained energy. A balanced diet that includes a variety of nutrient-dense food, including carbohydrates, proteins, fats, vitamins, and minerals, is key to supporting overall health and well-being.

3- **Body Regulators** – Vitamins, water, fruits, vegetables, and minerals keep the body running smoothly. Especially water is a good regulator. It helps every organ of the body to operate efficiently. It helps to unblock our physical machinery.

MINERALS AND VITAMINS

Minerals and vitamins are necessary nutrients that the body needs to function properly. They play crucial roles in various physiological processes, Including.

Metabolism, immune function, bone health, and many others. Here's some

Overview of minerals and vitamins:

Minerals – Minerals are inorganic substances that the body requires in relatively small amounts. They are necessary for building strong bones and teeth and maintaining them. Fluid balance, transmitting never impulses, and supporting various metabolic processes. Some key minerals include; - calcium, which is necessary for bones and teeth.

Health, muscle function, and nerve transmission.

Iron - Necessary for the production of hemoglobin, which carries oxygen in the blood.

Magnesium - Is involved in energy production, muscle function, and bone health.

Potassium - Is important for maintaining proper fluid balance, nerve function and Muscle contractions.

Zinc - Zinc supports immune function, wound healing, and DNA synthesis.

Vitamins

Vitamins are organic compounds that the body needs in small amounts to maintain normal physiological function. They play crucial roles in supporting growth vision, immune function, and various other processes. Vitamins are broadly categorized into two groups;

- **Fat-soluble vitamins:** Vitamins A, D, E, and K are fat-soluble vitamins, which means they are absorbed along with fats in the diet and stored in the body's fatty tissues. These vitamins are necessary for vision, bone health, antioxidant protection, and blood clotting.

- **Water-soluble vitamins:** Vitamins B family means vitamins B1, B2, B3, B6, and B12, and Vitamin C is a water-soluble vitamin and is not stored in the body to the same extent as fat-soluble vitamins. They play roles in energy production, red blood cell formation, nervous system function, and collagen synthesis.

It's important to consume a balanced diet that includes a variety of foods rich in essential minerals and vitamins to ensure optimal health.In some cases, diet supplements may be recommended to address specific deficiencies orHealth conditions. However, it's always best to obtain nutrients from whole foods Whenever possible.

PROTEIN IN DIET

Protein is an important macronutrient that plays a crucial role in the body. Here are some of the key reasons why protein is necessary in diet.

1- Muscle growth and repair - Protein provides the building blocks like amino acids Which are necessary for the growth, repair, and maintenance of muscle tissue. This is especially active or engaging in strength training.

2- Enzyme and hormone production - Proteins are required for the production of enzymes and hormones that regulate various bodily functions, such as metabolism, digestion, and immune response.

3- Cell structure and function -Proteins are integral to the structure and function of cells, tissues, and organs throughout the body.

4- Immune function - Certain proteins, such as antibodies, play a critical role in supporting the immune system and defending the body against infections and diseases.

5- Satiety and weight management - Protein-rich foods can help promote feelings of fullness and satiety, which may aid in weight management by reducing overall calorie intake.

6- Nutrient absorption - Protein is involved in the transportation and absorption of important nutrients, such as vitamins and minerals, within the body.

7- Energy production - while carbohydrates are the body's primary source of energy, protein can also be used as an energy source when necessary.

Overall, ensuring enough for what you need of protein is necessary for maintaining overall health, supporting physical performance, and promoting optimal body function.

Source of Protein

Protein can be obtained from a variety of food sources, including; -

1- **Animal-based sources** - Meat, pork, lamb, and game meats.

-Poultry: chicken, turkey, duck, and other fowl.

-Fish and seafood; -Salmon, tuna, shrimp, cod, and other types of fish and shellfish.

-Eggs; - Both the egg white and yolk are sources of protein.

2- **Dairy products** - Milk -Cow's milk, goat's milk, and other animal milk.

- Cheese; - Cheddar, mozzarella, Swiss, feta, and other types of cheese.

- Yogurt; - Greek yogurt, regular yogurt, and other dairy-based yogurts.

3- **Plant-based sources** - Legumes; - Beans, black beans, kidney Beans, chickpeas, lentils, and peas.

4- **Nuts and seeds** - Almonds, peanuts, walnuts, sunflower seeds, chia seeds, and flaxseeds.

5- **Soya Products** - Tofu, tempeh, edamame, and soya milk.

6- **Whole grains** - Quinoa, brown rice, barley, and whole wheat products.

7- **Other plant-based options** -Vegetables such as spinach, broccoli, and Brussels sprouts contain significant amounts of protein.

Plant-based meat substitutes; -Products made From soy, pea protein, or other plant-based ingredients can provide a protein source for those following a vegetarian or vegan diet.

It's important to consume a variety of protein sources to ensure that you get a good balance of essential amino acids and other nutrients. Different sources of protein also offer different nutritional benefits, so incorporating a mix of animal-based and plant-based protein sources into your diet can contribute to overall health and well-being.

Certainly! Protein powder has become a popular dietary supplement for many people looking to increase their protein intake, especially among athletes,

Bodybuilders and individuals following specific diets. Here are a few stories that Explain the role of protein powder in different dietary contexts.

1- Athlete's Recovery-After heavy workout, an athlete relies on protein to aid in Muscle recovery and repair. Consuming a protein shake or smoothie with Protein powder, they can quickly replenish their muscles with the necessary amino Acids to support recovery and growth.

2- Weight loss Journey- A person on a weight loss journey incorporates protein Powder into their diet plan to help manage hunger and maintain muscle mass While reducing overall calorie intake. They may use protein powder to create low-calorie, high-protein meal replacements or snacks to support their weight loss goals.

3- Vegetarian or Vegan diet -Individuals following a vegetarian or vegan diet may Use protein as a convenient way to ensure they meet their daily protein-derivedSources like pea, hemp, or brown rice can serve as an essential supplement to their diet, especially if they struggle to get enough protein from whole-food sources.

4- Busy Lifestyle- For someone with a hectic schedule, protein can be a convenient And a quick source of nutrition. They may use it to make a protein-packed Smoothie or shake as a meal replacement when they are short on time or need A portable option for on-the-go nutrition.

5- Muscle Building and Bodybuilding – Bodybuilders and strength athletes often Rely on protein powder as a key component of their muscle-building regimen. They may consume protein shakes immediately after workouts to promote Muscle protein synthesis and maximize growth. These points highlight the diverse ways in which protein can be integrated Into various dietary lifestyle and fitness goals. Whether it's for muscle recovery. Weight management, dietary restrictions, convenience, or muscle building, Protein offers a versatile and accessible means of meeting individual protein needs within the context of different dietary preferences and health objectives

WATER INTAKE OR DRINKING WATER

Water accounts for seventy percent of the human body's weight. Even our bones are forty percent water. All processes of life, humans, animals, and nature are dependent upon water. The evaporation of water from the skin is an essential factor in regulating the temperature of the body. The kidneys handle 170 to 180 quarts of water every day. Kidneys eliminate waste products of the body through urine and stool. When a person drinks a small amount of water, they will be sick. It is a favor to your kidneys to drink sufficient water.

What is the role of water in our life?

Water plays a crucial role in our lives in several ways-

Health- Drinking water is important for maintaining good health. It helps to prevent dehydration, which can lead to fatigue, headaches, and other health issues.

Dehydration- Water is essential for the proper functioning of our body. It helps to regulate body temperature, transport nutrients, and oxygen to cells, and remove waste products.

Cooking and food preparation- Water is used for cooking, cleaning fruits and vegetables, and food preparation in general.

Sanitation- Water is necessary for maintaining proper hygiene and sanitation. It is used for bathing, washing clothes, and cleaning our living spaces.

Agriculture- Water is essential for growing crops and raising livestock. It is used for irrigation and crop processing.

Overall, water is necessary for life and plays a big role in sustaining human health and the environment.

Purification of water

Pure water is good for health. It is safe for drinking. A great deal is said about the quality of water. We listen to many types of water: hard water, soft water, good water, bad water, and pure water. But pure water is safe for drinking. It contains no disease-producing germs or poisons.

Water purification is the process of removing contaminants and impurities from water to make it safe for consumption or other uses. There are several methods of water purification, each method designed for different types.

Filtration- This method involves passing water through a physical barrier, such as a filter or membrane, to remove particles, sediment, and larger impurities.

Distillation- Distillation involves heating water to create steam, which then comes back into liquid form, leaving behind contaminants that do not vaporize at the same temperature as water.

Chlorination- Chlorination is a chemical method in which chlorine or chlorine compounds are added to water to kill bacteria, viruses, and other harmful microorganisms.

Reverse Osmosis- This process involves forcing water through a semipermeable membrane to remove contaminants, including dissolved salts, minerals, and other impurities.

Boiling- Boiling water is a simple and effective method of water purification that kills most microorganisms and pathogens. This method uses everyone, poor or rich.

Chemical Treatment- Various chemicals, such as iodine or hydrogen peroxide, can kill harmful microorganisms. This treatment is under the supervision of an expert person.

The choice of water purification method depends on the specific contaminants present in the water and the desired level of purity. In many cases, a combination of different purification methods may be used to ensure that water is safe for consumption or other uses.

What is dehydration

Dehydration is when the body loses more water fluid than it takes in, leading to an imbalance in the body's water levels. This can result from a variety of factors, including excessive sweating, inadequate fluid intake, vomiting, diarrhea, or certain medical conditions.

When the body becomes dehydrated, it can disrupt normal physiological functions and lead to a range of symptoms, including;

1- Thirst

2- Dry mouth and dry skin

3- Fatigue and weakness

4- Dizziness or light-headedness

5- Dark yellow urine

6- Reduced urine output

7- Headaches

8- Confusion or irritability

9- Rapid heartbeat and breathing

10- Constipation

Severe dehydration can be life-threatening and may require medical intervention. It's important to address dehydration by replenishing lost fluids through drinking water, oral rehydration solutions, or, in severe cases, intravenous fluids administered by healthcare professionals.

Preventing dehydration involves maintaining a proper balance of fluid intake and output, especially during hot weather, physical activity, illness, or other situations that increase the risk of fluid loss. Staying hydrated is compulsory for overall health and well-being.

How much and When to Drink Water

The amount of water a person needs to drink water can vary depending on factors such as age, gender, activity level, and overall health. However, a general guideline is to aim for about 8-10 cups or glasses of water per day for most adults. This can come from a combination of water, other beverages, and water-rich foods.

It is important to listen to your body's signals for thirst and to drink water throughout the day. Some people may need more water, especially if they are physically active, live in a hot climate, or are experiencing illness or pregnancy.

In terms of drinking water -

1- Upon Walking - Drinking a glass of water in the morning can help you rehydrate your body after a night's sleep and kickstart your metabolism.

2- Throughout the day; - Sip water regularly throughout the day to maintain hydration. Carry a reusable water bottle with you to make it easier to stay hydrated.

3- Before meals; -Drinking water before meals can help you with digestion and may also help prevent overeating.

4- During physical activity - Drinking water before, during, and after exercise to replace fluids lost through sweating.

5- When feeling thirsty is a signal that your body needs more fluids, so be sure to drink water when you feel thirsty.

It's important to note that individual hydration needs can vary, so it's best to pay attention to your body's signals and adjust your fluid intake accordingly. If you have specific health concerns or conditions that affect your fluid balance, it's a good idea to consult with a healthcare expert for personalized recommendations.

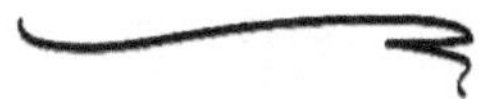

PART 4: WORKING HABITS

WHY WORKING HABITS?

Creating good working habits can help you become more productive, focused, and efficient in your professional or personal endeavors. Working habits can vary widely from person to person, but here are some tips for developing effective working habits.

Set Clear Goals; - Define specific, achievable goals for your work. Having a clear understanding of what you want to accomplish will help you stay motivated and focused.

Prioritize Task: Identify the most important and urgent tasks and prioritize them. This will help you allocate your time and energy effectively.

Create Routine; -Establish a daily or weekly routine that includes dedicated time for work, breaks, and other activities. Consistency can help you get into a productive mindset and make it easier to manage your workload.

Time Management; -Use time management techniques such as the Pomodoro technique [working in focused intervals with short breaks] or time blocking, allocating specific time slots for different tasks to make the most of your work hours.

Minimize Distractions; -Identify and minimize potential distractions in your work environment. This could include turning off notifications, finding a quiet workspace, or using tools to block distracting websites or apps.

Reflect and Adjust: Regularly evaluate your work habits and productivity levels.

Identify areas for improvement and make adjustments as needed to optimize your workflow.

Self-Care; -Prioritize self-care practices such as exercise, adequate sleep, and healthy eating habits. Taking care of your physical and mental well-being can have a positive impact on your work performance.

Celebrate Achievements; -Acknowledge and celebrate your accomplishments, no matter how small. This can help reinforce positive working habits and motivate you to continue making progress.

By incorporating these strategies into your daily routine, you can develop effective working habits that support your professional and personal growth in your life.

These four habits help you keep fit and active every time;

1- Gardening

2- Read good books

3- Controle your weight

4- Reduce stress

GARDENING

Gardening is the practice of cultivating and nurturing plants, flowers, fruits, vegetables, or other types of vegetation in a designated area such as a garden, yard, or plot of land. It involves a range of activities, including planting, watering, weeding, fertilizing, and caring for plants to promote their growth and health. This habit makes a pleasure your inner side. Gardening can be pursued for various purposes, like this;

To look beautiful: Many people do gardening to create visually appealing and beautiful outdoor spaces, such as flower gardens, ornamental landscapes, or themed gardens.

Here is a story of my friends who lived in Canada. They are a very charming couple at a young age. Their family was a joint family in Canada, but after a few years, they lived separately from their family because of some family problems. When they live Separately, they feel alone and sad. One day, I suggest they be involved in an agricultural fair that a big company, almond growing, organizes. They participate in this fair as a gust, but they feel very happy and excited after that fair. They are entrusted to grow some flowers and vegetables in their empty plot. Now they are very happy because of gardening. They told me one day that every person who passed the way of my house can't leave without saying Wow.

For food production; -Gardner's may grow fruits, vegetables, herbs, and other edible plants to harvest fresh produce for consumption. This can contribute to a sustainable and healthy lifestyle.

Environmental Funding; -Gardening can involve the cultivation of native plants, Trees and shrubs to support local ecosystems and wildlife habitats. It can also Contribute to environmental conservation efforts.

Therapeutic Benefits; -For some individuals, gardening serves as a therapeutic and stress-relieving activity that promotes relaxation, mindfulness, and a connection to nature.

Gardening practices can vary widely based on factors such as climate, soil type, available space, and personal preferences. It can be pursued on a small scale in containers or raised beds or on a larger scale in expansive gardens or agricultural plots.

Overall, gardening is a versatile and rewarding activity that allows individuals to engage with nature, promote sustainability, and enjoy the beauty and bounty of plant life.

READ GOOD BOOKS

Book reading is one of the best choices for every intelligent person. When you start reading books, you want to do only what is necessary. Your body and mind command in your hand, because books are very good friend of you. Here are some tips to help you start the habit of book reading.

Set a specific time for reading; -Choose a time of the day when you can dedicate at least 20-30 minutes to reading. This could be in the morning, during your lunch break, or before bed.

Create a comfortable spot where you can read without distractions. Make it cozy with a comfortable chair, good lighting, and a warm blanket if needed.

Start with shorter books or articles you're new to reading. Start with shorter books or articles that interest you. This will help you build momentum and confidence.

Set a reading goal; -Set a realistic goal for the number of books that you want to read in a month or year. This can motivate you to stay consistent with your reading habits.

Limit your screen time- Reduce your screen time, especially on electronic devices, to create more time for reading.

Join a book club- Joining a book club or reading group can provide accountability and motivation to keep reading regularly.

Make it enjoyable- Choose books that you are genuinely interested in and enjoy reading. Don't force yourself to read something you are not enjoying.

Keep track of your progress- Consider keeping a reading journal or using a reading to track the books you have read and set new reading goals.

Remember that building a habit takes time and consistency, so be patient with yourself as you work on establishing a regular reading routine.

CONTROL YOUR WEIGHT

Overweight problems are everywhere in the world. Everyone knows what diseases could come with obesity, but we do not take care of them. When the obesity problem increases, so do we run here and there to control our weight, but we are not ready to change our bad lifestyle.

There are the diseases name that can be with obesity:

- Type 2 diabetes

- High blood pressure

- Heart disease

- Stroke

- Certain types of cancer [such as breast, colon, and kidney]

- Sleep apnoea

- Osteoarthritis

- Fatty liver disease

- Kidney stone and disease

- Gallbladder disease

These are the most common illnesses associated with being overweight. It's important to note that overweight can also contribute to a range of other health issues, including mental health conditions such as depression and anxiety. It's always best to continue to exercise before we get overweight.

Controlling body weight involves a combination of healthy eating, regular physical activity, and lifestyle.

Eat a balanced diet and always focus on consuming a variety of nutrient-dense foods such as fruits, vegetables, whole grains, lean protein, and healthy fats. Limit your intake of processed food, sugary snacks, and high-calorie beverages.

Monitor your calorie intake- Keep track of the calories that you consume and ensure that you are not consistently consuming daily or more calories than your body needs.

REDUCE STRESS

Stress is a natural response to challenging or threatening situations. It is the body's way of reacting to a demand or pressure and can be triggered by various factors, such as work, relationships, financial issues, or major life changes. When faced with stress, the body releases hormones like adrenaline and cortisol, which can lead to physical, emotional, and mental changes.

Stress can manifest in different ways, including physical symptoms like headaches, muscle tension, and stomach problems, as well as emotional symptoms like anxiety, irritability, and feeling overwhelmed. Prolonged or chronic stress can have negative effects on overall health, including an increased risk for conditions like heart disease, depression, and anxiety disorders.

Reason of stress

Many people take unnecessary tension. If you have some time for mental activity, you feel happy for the whole day and your whole life. Stress can make you upset. The students struggling with academic pressure start to feel stressed. Here is a story of a student who is an excellent student but is always under stress.

Mandy was a high school student who had always been an excellent student. However, as he entered his senior year, the pressure to excel academically became overwhelming. He spends long hours in study but does not participate in any other activity. When his physical education teacher asked him to be involved in any other co-curricular activity, he ignored the teacher's point. He felt pressured to secure a scholarship for college or university. As a result, Mandy began experiencing anxiety attacks, difficulty concentrating, and a decline in his overall mental health.

With the support of his parents and the help of his school physical education teacher, Mandy learned to set realistic goals, prioritize self-care, and seek help when he needed it. When he starts participating in the playground, he feels better than before. By managing his workload more effectively and seeking support, he was able to reduce his stress levels and improve his overall well-being.

Stress is not the only problem of students; rather, the person working in each field is in stress. I met a lady named Sarah. She was a successful executive at a large corporation. She was constantly under pressure to meet deadlines, attend meetings, and manage her team. Her job demanded long hours and frequent travel. She never has some time for her baby and her family. Over time, the stress of her job began to take a toll on her health. She experienced frequent headaches, insomnia, and irritability.

Eventually, Sarah realized that she needed to make some changes in her life to manage her stress better. She started delegating more tasks at work start, self-care, and spending more quality time with her child and her family. By making these adjustments, she was able to regain a sense of balance and reduce the impact of stress on her good health.

The world is full of such stories, but the question is how to avoid them. By taking some free time in your busy life and using it properly when working, you avoid stress. It can affect individuals in different aspects of their lives, and it is important to find healthy ways to manage it.

DISCLAIMER

This book is for informational purposes only. Readers acknowledge that the author does not render legal, financial, medical, or professional advice. The content within this book has been derived from various sources. Please consult a licensed professional before attempting any techniques outlined in this book.

By reading this document, the reader agrees that under no circumstances is the author responsible for any direct or indirect losses incurred as a result of the use of the information contained within this document, including but not limited to errors, omissions, or inaccuracies. Adherence to all applicable laws and regulations, including international, federal, state, and local governing professional licensing, business practices, advertising, and all other jurisdictions, is the sole responsibility of the purchaser or reader. Neither the author nor the publisher assumes any responsibility or liability whatsoever on behalf of the purchaser or reader of these materials. Any perceived slight of any individual or organization is purely unintentional.

MAY I ASK YOU A FAVOR?

At the outset, I want to give you a big thanks for reading this book. You could have chosen any other book, but you took mine, and I appreciate this. I hope you have at least a few actionable insights that will positively impact your daily life.

Can I ask for 30 seconds more of your time?

I'd love it if you could leave a review of the book. That will help me grow my readership by encouraging folks to take a chance on my books.

Keeping it straight - reviews are the lifeblood of any author.

It will take less than a minute of your time but will tremendously help me reach out to more people. Kindly provide your review at the store you bought this book from. And I'd love to see your review. Thanks for your support.

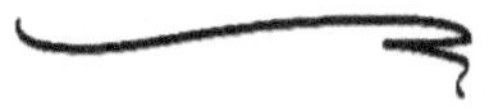